THE EDGAR CAYCE WAY OF OVERCOMING MULTIPLE SCLEROSIS: VIBRATORY MEDICINE

By

Dr. Dudley Delany

Foreword By
Dr. C. Norman Shealy

Fourth Edition

Printed in the United States of America.

Published by: Meridian Publications
P.O. Box 7987
Hampton, VA 23666

Publisher's Cataloging in Publication Data:

Delany, Dudley, 1940-

The Edgar Cayce Way of Overcoming Multiple Sclerosis: Vibratory Medicine/by Dr. Dudley Delany, 4th ed.

Library of Congress Catalog Card
Number: 97-93411
120 p.: ill.; 22 cm.
Includes appendix, bibliography, and index.
ISBN-0-9657903-3-9 (pbk.): $10.95

1. Cayce, Edgar, 1877-1945
2. Multiple sclerosis–alternative treatment.

I. Title.

D337 6[redacted]

DEDICATION

This book is affectionately dedicated to the patients and staff on the spinal cord injury ward of the V.A. Medical Center in Hampton, Virginia.

IMPORTANT NOTE TO READERS WITH MS

It is essential that the treatment recommendations contained in this publication be implemented with the knowledge, consent, and cooperation of your attending physician, so that he or she can propose any appropriate modifications, closely monitor your progress, adjust your medication schedule if necessary, intervene as needed with helpful advice and suggestions, and document whatever results may be obtained. In addition, it is possible that your experience with vibratory medicine may inspire him or her to undertake *desperately* needed research in a field that has the potential of bringing health, help, and healing to *millions*. For vibratory medicine has been found to be effective in treating not only multiple sclerosis, but many other conditions as well, some of which (such as muscular dystrophy and Lou Gehrig's disease) are, on the whole, even more serious and debilitating than MS.

FOREWORD

Like Dr. Delany, I have been a student of Edgar Cayce for many years. Much of the health advice that Cayce gave has been shown to be effective in a variety of situations. This book is, however, to my knowledge, the first documentation of continuing benefit from the very simple and safe treatments Cayce proposed well over 50 years ago.

Modern conventional medicine has relatively little to offer individuals with MS. Those medications currently in use to treat it carry a number of undesirable "side effects" or complications, and certainly are not curative.

If I had MS, I hope that I would have the wisdom, no matter what else I might do, to incorporate the Cayce suggestions.

The extensive comments about good nutrition in MS are themselves worthy of considerable study.

You have nothing to lose following the program that Dr. Delany has outlined based on the Cayce material, but you potentially have everything to gain. Indeed, there is a great deal to celebrate and a lot to recommend in following the advice in this book.

C. Norman Shealy, M.D., Ph.D.
Founder, Shealy Institute for
Comprehensive Health Care
Springfield, MO 65803-4400

PREFACE

Based on the work of the late Edgar Cayce, *vibratory medicine is a very mild form of electrotherapy which treats human ills by administering – in a painless and non-invasive manner – the essential essence or "vibration" of certain substances having medicinal properties.* It is a way of administering substances which are relatively *toxic* to the body (like *gold* in the treatment of rheumatoid arthritis) *without* adverse effects; it is a way of administering substances in which the body may be *deficient* (like *iron* in the treatment of anemia) *without* using food supplements; it is a way of administering substances to which the body may be *allergic* (like *iodine* in the treatment of goiter) *without* causing allergic reactions. It represents a totally new idea, a totally new concept, a totally new approach to administering selected medicinal agents, and it has the potential of *revolutionizing* medicine.

At least two devices currently exist to accomplish the goals of vibratory medicine, the "radial appliance" and the "wet cell battery."

These pages relate the manner in which I and others used vibratory medicine to overcome *multiple sclerosis*, a chronic, sometimes disabling neurological disorder of unknown cause that afflicts an estimated 350,000 to 500,000 Americans.

It is hoped that this publication will be a blessing, a comfort, and an encouragement to those who seek an "alternative approach" to defeating this disturbing, sometimes devastating disease for which, at the present time, medical science has no cure.

Dudley Delany, R.N., M.A., D.C.
Hampton, Virginia

TABLE OF CONTENTS

CHAPTER 1

THE EDGAR CAYCE LEGACY

Edgar Cayce was born near Hopkinsville, Kentucky, in 1877. A man of humble means and with very little formal education, he became a photographer, married a delicate, sensitive woman, and eventually fathered three boys. A devout Christian, he became a Sunday School teacher, and read the Bible through once for every year of his life. His hobbies included fishing, bowling, golf, and playing cards.

What really set Edgar Cayce apart from the mass of humanity was the fact that, at the age of thirteen, he encountered an *angel* who asked him what he *most* wanted in life. The young man replied that he wanted to *help* people, especially children. At the age of twenty-one, Edgar Cayce developed the astounding ability to enter a self-induced hypnotic trance in which he could *diagnose illnesses* and *prescribe treatments* for individuals he had not only never seen before, but who might perhaps be thousands of miles away.

These trance discourses came to be known as "readings," and they proved to be so helpful to so many that it was decided early on to record, preserve, and study them.

When Edgar Cayce died in 1945, he left a legacy of over 14,000 readings, all of which are on file (and also on CD-ROM computer disc) at the Association for Research and Enlightenment, 67th Street and Atlantic Avenue, Virginia Beach, VA 23451. The A.R.E. makes available to any interested party not only the readings, but also the many books, articles, audio cassettes, and video presentations based on them. It also publishes two bi-monthly magazines, *Venture Inward* and *The New Millennium,* both of which discuss the readings and various related topics.

While some of the readings deal with dream analysis, Bible interpretation, future events, and other subjects, the majority address most of the ills to which flesh is heir.

Included in those ills were numerous health problems for which the readings recommended the "vibratory" administration of various substances using either the radial appliance or the wet cell battery. The design, construction, operation, maintenance, care, and use of these devices are based solely on information provided by the readings.

Unlike the light bulb and the phonograph, the appliances were not "invented." Rather, they were *given* – as a *gift* to the world – through a sleeping photographer – by some "source" that apparently has great wisdom, great compassion, and great love for a suffering and afflicted humanity.

They that wait upon the LORD shall renew their strength; they shall mount up with wings as eagles; they shall run and not be weary; and they shall walk, and not faint.

Isaiah 40:31

CHAPTER 2

THE RADIAL APPLIANCE

INTRODUCTION

The radial appliance (also referred to as the impedance device, the radio-active appliance, and the dry cell) was recommended in over 900 readings in the treatment of such conditions as nervous tension, poor circulation, insomnia, vaginitis, neurasthenia, debilitation, hypertension, migraine headaches, psoriasis, deafness, obesity, tic douloureux, tuberculosis, leukemia, and sterility.

CONSTRUCTION DETAILS

Although minor variations exist between models of different manufacturers, in general, the appliance consists of a metal container (2" X 2-1/4" X 6-1/2") containing two high-carbon-content rectangular steel rods (each 1/4" X 1/2" X 5") separated by two pieces of glass (each 1/16" X 1/2" X 5") and surrounded on four sides by four pieces of carbon (two are 1/4" X 1/2" X 5" and two are 1/4" X 1-3/16" X 5"). This carbon-steel-glass "sandwich" is wrapped like a cocoon in masking tape and immersed in charcoal particles. Each steel rod attaches to a terminal on the outside of the appliance.

The appliance also comes equipped with a round, slightly concave copper electrode (1" in diameter), a round, slightly concave nickel electrode (2-1/2" in diameter), a four-ounce-capacity "solution jar" containing a loop (1/8" in diameter) made of nickel in the shape of a "U" (although other shapes are available, *use only this one*), and appropriate connecting wire (see Figure 1).

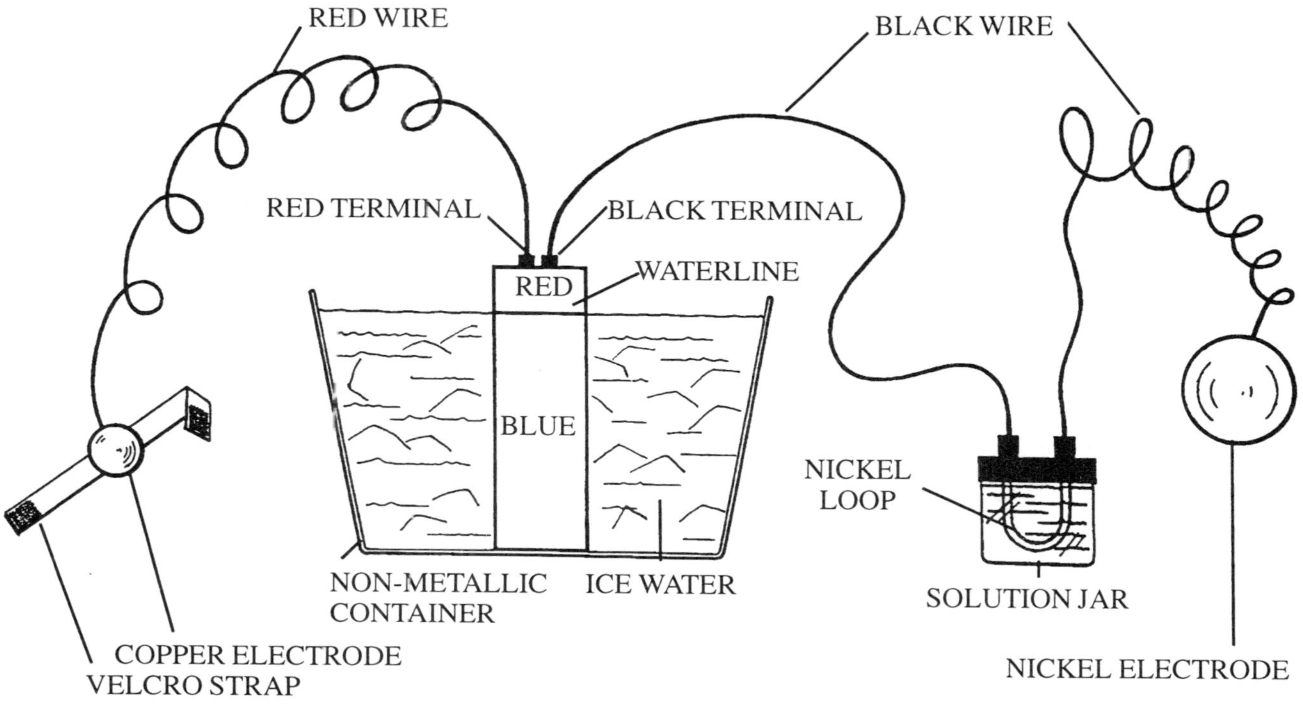

FIGURE 1: RADIAL APPLIANCE WITH SOLUTION JAR.

HOW THE RADIAL APPLIANCE IS USED

There are *two* ways in which the radial appliance may be utilized: (1) *without* the solution jar, and (2) *with* the solution jar.

Use of the appliance *without* the solution jar is intended mainly to promote relaxation, improve circulation, and balance the body mentally, physically, and spiritually. For a discussion of how the appliance is connected to the body and utilized in this way, the interested reader is referred to literature available from the parties listed in the Appendix.

Use of the appliance *with* the solution jar is intended mainly to introduce into the body the essential essence or vibration of some particular substance (such as iodine, silver, iron, quinine, or gold) *without* introducing the actual substance itself. One might liken it to introducing the scent of a rose but not the rose itself, or the music of a violin but not the violin itself, or the warmth and glow of a lighted candle but not the candle itself. This task is accomplished (as can be seen in Figure 1) by routing the flow of energy from the *black* (normally negative) terminal on the appliance *through the solution jar*, where the vibration of the desired substance is acquired. Leaving the solution jar, the energy is then deposited on the nickel electrode (which is often placed on the abdomen near the navel). It then enters and flows through the body, is collected by the copper electrode (which is often attached to the wrist or ankle), and returned to the appliance via the *red* (normally positive) terminal.

Although a "subtle" energy component may also be involved, the nature of this energy is a naturally occurring form of electricity produced by the body itself. The appliance merely induces and modulates its flow.

The substance to be placed in the solution jar varies depending on the condition to be treated. The one most frequently recommended, however, was *gold* (in the form of a dilute solution of gold chloride). The readings stated that the vibratory administration of gold would help rejuvenate *any* organ that was "delinquent" in its action. How that occurs, and what connection gold has with tissue growth, repair, healing, and regeneration is not clear.

STEPS IN OPERATING THE APPLIANCE

In setting up and using the radial appliance,

(1) change the solution in the jar after *fifteen* uses;

(2) cover the solution jar with the *bare* lid when not using the appliance;

(3) keep the solution jar in a *dark* place when not in use;

(4) never allow the solution jar to come into direct contact with sunlight;

(5) before use, carefully sand and polish the loop and the rim and cup of both electrodes with 600 grit sandpaper (giving them a final wipe with tissue paper);

(6) always use a protective ("dust") mask when sanding (available at most hardware stores and pharmacies or by calling 1-800-BEDFORD);

(7) before use, place the appliance into a suitable non-metallic container (such as a plastic paint pail); fill the container with *ice* to the waterline on the appliance; then fill the container with *water* to the waterline;

(8) never allow water to come up over the top of the appliance or to cover the attached wiring;

(9) allow the appliance to cool down in the ice water *twenty minutes* before attachment to the body;

(10) *five minutes* before attaching the appliance to the body, put the loop into the solution jar and screw down the lid; connect the solution jar to the *black terminal* on the appliance; then connect the nickel electrode to the solution jar;

(11) begin your session on the appliance by assuming a relaxed, comfortable reclining position in a location free from distractions or disturbances; connect the

copper electrode to the *red terminal* on the appliance; then apply the copper electrode to the body;

(12) if applying the copper electrode to an extremity, use the Velcro strap to hold it in place (make the strap loose enough so as not to impede circulation);

(13) if applying the copper electrode elsewhere, secure it with adhesive tape or other suitable means;

(14) after the copper electrode has been properly situated, apply the nickel electrode, securing it with adhesive tape or other expedient;

(15) always be sure to apply the copper electrode *first*;

(16) insure that both electrodes lie *flat* against the skin;

(17) maintain each session for a period of *thirty minutes*;

(18) occupy your time on the appliance in prayer, meditation, and/or reading the Bible or other inspirational literature;

(19) when your session is over, remove the nickel and then the copper electrode from the body; disconnect the electrodes from the appliance; disconnect the black wiring from the solution jar; dry off the loop and carefully sand and polish it

with 600 grit sandpaper (giving it a final wipe with tissue paper); remove the appliance from the ice water, dry it off, and place it in the sun; then carefully sand and polish the rim and cup of both electrodes with 600 grit sandpaper (giving them a final wipe with tissue paper);

(20) keep the appliance from the elements if placed in the sun *outdoors*;

(21) never allow the electrodes and their associated wiring to touch, whether attached to the appliance or not;

(22) never allow the appliance to come into contact with anything metallic;

(23) if attempting to administer more than one substance vibratorially, for each solution, provide a separate jar, loop, and nickel electrode; and

(24) patiently and persistently persevere in the use of the appliance.

CHAPTER 3

THE WET CELL BATTERY

INTRODUCTION

The wet cell battery (also known as the wet cell appliance) was recommended in about 975 readings in the treatment of such conditions as Down's syndrome, spinal cord injuries, scleroderma, stroke, alcoholism, major depression, schizophrenia, color blindness, Parkinson's disease, muscular dystrophy, Lou Gehrig's disease, Alzheimer's disease, rheumatoid arthritis, cancer, polio, and multiple sclerosis.

CONSTRUCTION DETAILS

There are currently two types of wet cell batteries on the market, one with short (8" to 10") poles, and one with long (14" to 16") poles. In my opinion, insofar as treating multiple sclerosis is concerned, either model will do nicely. The short pole version is illustrated in Figure 1. The long pole version is similar in design and operation, but is taller and more slender in appearance.

What we have in Figure 1 is essentially the configuration of a simple wet cell battery, consisting of two cylindrical rods or "poles," each measuring 1/2" in diameter and between 8" and 10" long, one made of copper and the other of nickel, suspended in an electrolytic solution. The container holds two gallons and has a matching lid (both are made of non-metallic material).

On top of each pole is a terminal. The one attached to the copper pole is *red* and represents the *positive* side of the battery. The one attached to the nickel pole is *black* and represents the *negative* side.

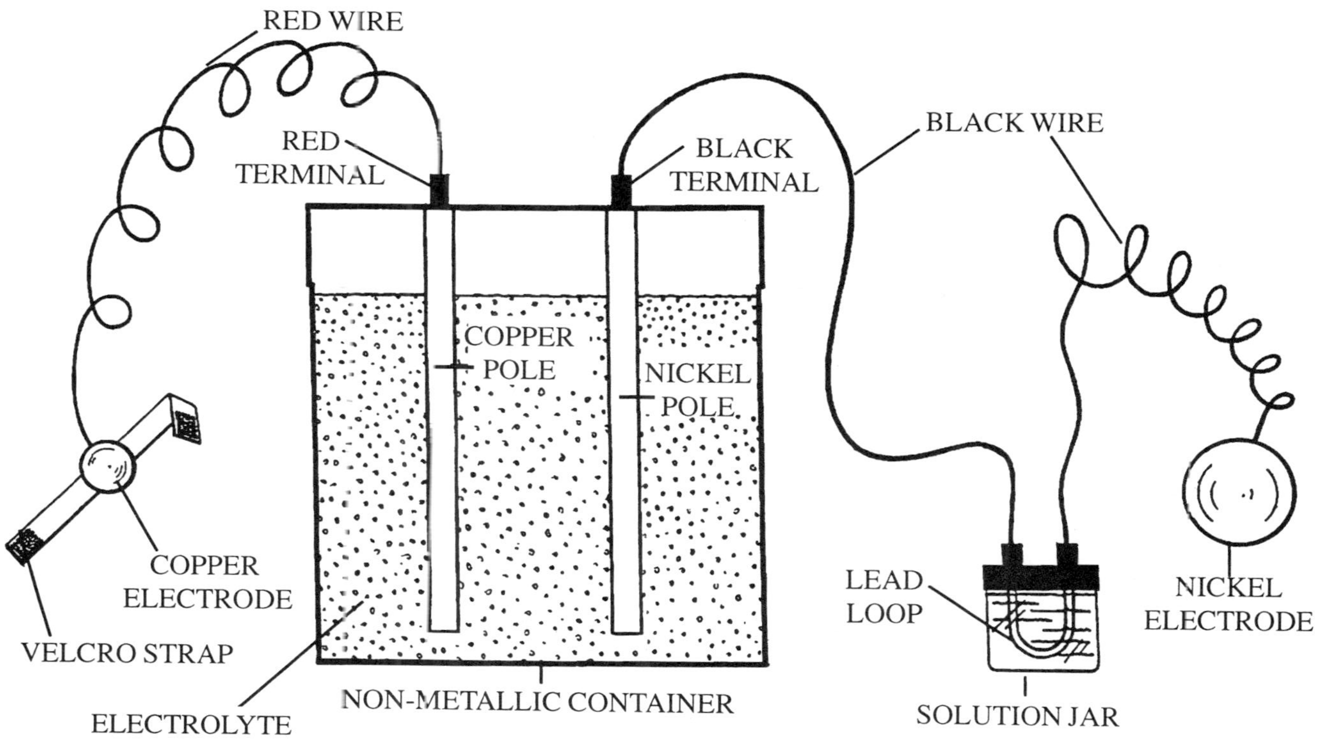

FIGURE 1: WET CELL BATTERY (SHORT POLE TYPE)

The wet cell battery comes equipped with a round, slightly concave copper electrode (1" in diameter), a round, slightly concave nickel electrode (2-1/2" in diameter), a four-ounce-capacity solution jar containing a loop made of hollow lead tubing (3/16" in diameter) in the shape of a "U" (although other shapes are available, *use only this one*), and appropriate connecting wire.

ELECTROLYTE PREPARATION

The electrolyte is prepared by pouring 1-1/2 gallons of distilled water into the container, and adding and mixing (with a wooden stick or utensil) in the order named:

(1) 1-1/2 pounds of copper sulfate,
(2) 4 ounces of sulfuric acid (25% solution),
(3) 5.3 grams of zinc particles, and
(4) 1/2 pound of willow charcoal.

THE ZINC CONTROVERSY

The exact amount of zinc necessary in the electrolyte is currently a subject of much debate among appliance manufacturers. The figure shown above (and those given in Chapter 4) are based on certain *MS readings* which specify that a "regular" charge requires 3 drams (5.3 grams), and that a "double strength" charge requires 6 drams (10.6 grams) of zinc.

HOW THE WET CELL BATTERY IS USED

The wet cell battery is usually utilized *with* the solution jar. Its primary function, therefore, is the vibratory administration of various medicinal agents.

As can be seen in Figure 1, energy flows from the *black* (negative) terminal on the appliance *through the solution jar*, where the vibration of the desired substance is acquired. It is then deposited on the nickel electrode (which is often placed on the abdomen near the navel), flows through the body, is collected by the copper electrode (which is often placed on a particular spinal vertebra), and returned to the appliance via the *red* (positive) terminal.

The nature of this energy is frankly electrical (although a subtle energy component may also be involved) and it can easily be measured with the appropriate instruments. Typically, the wet cell battery develops between 20 and 35 millivolts of electrical potential.

In comparison to the radial appliance, there is very little mystery surrounding the wet cell battery – everything is out in the open; we learn about batteries in school; and we use them to start our cars, power our flashlights, etc.

STEPS IN OPERATING THE WET CELL

In setting up and using the wet cell battery,

(1) let the electrolyte mix and dissolve for 24 hours after preparation before using the appliance;

(2) place the appliance where it need not be moved to utilize it;

(3) change the solution in the solution jar after *fifteen* uses;

(4) cover the solution jar with the *bare* lid when not using the appliance;

(5) keep the solution jar in a *dark* place when not in use;

(6) never allow the solution jar to come into direct contact with sunlight;

(7) before use, carefully sand and polish the loop and the rim and cup of both electrodes with 600 grit sandpaper (giving them a final wipe with tissue paper);

(8) always use a protective (dust) mask when sanding (and also when doing dusty housework);

(9) *twenty minutes* before the attachment of the wet cell to the body, put the loop into the solution jar and screw down the lid; connect the solution jar to the *black terminal* on the appliance; connect the nickel electrode to the solution jar; then connect the copper electrode to the *red terminal* on the appliance;

(10) begin your session on the wet cell by assuming a relaxed, comfortable reclining position in a location free from distractions or disturbances; then apply the copper electrode to the body;

(11) if applying the copper electrode to an extremity, use the Velcro strap to hold it in place (make the strap loose enough so as not to impede circulation);

(12) if applying the copper electrode elsewhere, secure it with adhesive tape or other suitable means;

(13) after the copper electrode has been properly situated, apply the nickel electrode, securing it with adhesive tape or other expedient;

(14) always be sure to apply the copper electrode *first*;

(15) insure that both electrodes lie *flat* against the skin;

(16) maintain each session for a period of *thirty minutes*;

(17) occupy your time on the wet cell in prayer, meditation, and/or reading the Bible or other inspirational literature;

(18) when your session is over, remove the nickel and then the copper electrode from the body; disconnect the electrodes from the appliance; disconnect the black wiring from the solution jar; dry off the loop, and carefully sand and polish it

with 600 grit sandpaper (giving it a final wipe with tissue paper); then carefully sand and polish the rim and cup of both electrodes with 600 grit sandpaper (giving them a final wipe with tissue paper);

(19) place the loop, wiring, and electrodes in the sun between sessions;

(20) never allow the electrodes and their associated wiring to touch, whether attached to the appliance or not;

(21) after *thirty* uses, discard the electrolyte; clean out and dry the container; remove all accumulations from the poles with sandpaper, a wire brush, and, if necessary, a file (giving them a final wipe with tissue paper); then store the appliance in a safe place until it is time to prepare the electrolyte for the next series of treatments;

(22) if attempting to administer more than one substance vibratorially, for each solution, provide a separate jar, loop, and nickel electrode; and

(23) patiently and persistently persevere in the use of the appliance.

CHAPTER 4

WHAT THE READINGS SAY ABOUT MULTIPLE SCLEROSIS

Edgar Cayce gave scores of readings for dozens of persons who appeared to be suffering from multiple sclerosis. He also gave one reading (907-1) for a physician who sought specific information on its cause and treatment. Most of these readings are reproduced in the A.R.E. Circulating Files on MS (available by calling 1-800-333-4499).

THE CAUSE AND TREATMENT OF MULTIPLE SCLEROSIS

The readings recognized many types of MS, but cited the usual cause as "glands" – especially those pertaining to digestion and assimilation.

In what is apparently the most common scenario, a glandular disturbance involving the *liver* (in association with the spleen, pancreas, and possibly other organs) leads to the inadequate absorption, distribution, and/or utilization of the trace amounts of *gold* normally present in the diet. Without sufficient quantities of gold in the system, certain neurotrophic glands (possibly unicellular) located in various segments of the spine – including the sacrum and coccyx (tail bone) – become incapable of secreting that which is necessary to maintain the structural and functional integrity of nerve cells. The result is a neurodestructive process that begins in the lower portion of the spinal cord and gradually progresses upward to the brain. In males, the lack of gold also hinders the normal production of sperm cells, causing a measure of sterility. This whole sequence of events is based on a congenital predisposition, and may be precipitated by such factors as nutritional deficiencies (particularly of gold, silver, iodine, and iron), injuries to the spine, vertebral subluxations, liver congestion, local or systemic infections, negative attitudes and/or emotions, environmental toxins, calcium chloride ingestion, and childbearing. The congenital predisposition may be due to heredity, adverse conditions surrounding conception, or both.

The usual treatment involved instilling gold into the body vibratorially by means of the wet cell. To facilitate the healing process, massage therapy (aimed primarily at stimulating and energizing nerves) and close attention to diet were also frequently recommended.

TREATING MULTIPLE SCLEROSIS WITH THE WET CELL BATTERY

The specifics of using the wet cell battery in the treatment of MS generally varied somewhat from case to case, but one effective approach might be to:

(1) employ the device in continuous cycles of 30 days with a five day "rest" interval between each cycle;
(2) use a three ounce solution of gold chloride (available from the suppliers listed in the Appendix) in the solution jar (in a concentration of one grain of gold chloride per ounce of distilled water);
(3) apply the copper electrode alternately to the *ninth dorsal* vertebra one day, and to the *fourth lumbar* vertebra the next day; and
(4) always place the nickel electrode on the abdomen slightly above and to the right of the navel (as illustrated on page 49).

In addition to the sacrum and coccyx, the vertebral column consists of seven cervical (neck) vertebrae, twelve dorsal (thoracic) vertebrae, and five lumbar (low back) vertebrae.

The row of "bumps" you see running up and down the middle of a person's back are the *spinous processes* (rearmost projections) of the vertebrae.

To locate the *fourth lumbar* vertebra, draw an imaginary line across the small of the back between the tops of the iliac crests. It should intersect the vertebral column at about the level of the fourth lumbar vertebra. The spinous process of this vertebra is the alternate site for placing the copper electrode.

The largest projection at the base of the back of the neck is usually the spinous process of the seventh cervical vertebra. Just below it is the spinous process of the first dorsal vertebra.

To locate the *ninth dorsal* vertebra, one method is to count down nine bumps from the first dorsal vertebra. Depending on the physique of the person with whom you are working, however, that method may be difficult or impossible. An alternate method is to have the person sit erect. Draw an imaginary line between the lower tips of the scapulae (shoulder blades). It should intersect the vertebral column at about the level of the seventh dorsal vertebra. Count down two bumps and you should be at the level of ninth dorsal vertebra. The copper electrode should be placed initially on the spinous process of this vertebra.

MASSAGE IN THE TREATMENT OF MULTIPLE SCLEROSIS

After each session on the wet cell battery, it is suggested that massage therapy be administered (preferably on a massage table) as follows:

(1) use Aura Glow (available from the Heritage Store listed in the Appendix) or a mixture of equal amounts of cold-pressed peanut oil and virgin olive oil;

(2) massage the oil (as much as the body will absorb) into the skin beginning at the base of the skull and working down the neck and back on both sides of the spine, across the lumbar and sacral areas, into the gluteal muscles, and down both legs to the feet and toes;

(3) massage the shoulders, arms, and hands;

(4) use mostly a circular or rotary motion; and

(5) maintain each session for a period of thirty minutes.

DIET IN THE TREATMENT OF MULTIPLE SCLEROSIS

It is recommended that you

(1) avoid alcoholic beverages;

(2) avoid ingesting any products containing caffeine (found in coffee, tea, chocolate, and many soft drinks);

(3) avoid ingesting anything containing white sugar (as a substitute, the readings suggest using honey, beet sugar, brown sugar, or saccharin);

(4) avoid smoked foods;
(5) avoid foods containing nitrates, nitrites, benzoate of soda, calcium chloride, MSG, and other chemical additives and preservatives;
(6) never eat fried food of any kind;
(7) never eat pork (except for some occasional very crisp bacon);
(8) never drink carbonated beverages;
(9) do not eat beef;
(10) eat *ocean* fish often (also good occasionally are poultry, lamb, and liver);
(11) avoid starchy foods like rice, potatoes, and pasta;
(12) fruits, vegetables, and their juices are very good;
(13) avoid spicy foods;
(14) eat only breads and cereals of the *whole grain* variety;
(15) eat quantities of lettuce every day (it acts as a blood purifier);
(16) do not combine whole grain cereals or dairy products with citrus fruit or citrus fruit juices at the same meal;
(17) salads (preferably gelatin) made with grated or chopped *raw* carrots, lettuce, celery, watercress, radishes, onions, tomatoes, and/or *cooked* beets are excellent;
(18) except for small quantities of butter, avoid products high in saturated (animal) fat, such as whole milk and hard cheese (skim milk, yogurt, and cottage cheese are alright);

(19) in regard to eggs, eat only the *yolks*, and make sure they are thoroughly cooked;
(20) do not eat if you are excessively fatigued, excited, angry, or upset;
(21) take a few alfalfa and a few dcsiccated liver tablets with each meal;
(22) never ingest anything prepared or stored in aluminum;
(23) eat a few almonds every day;
(24) use little or no salt;
(25) avoid *raw* apples unless you are on the apple cleansing diet (see Question 8 on page 70);
(26) take, after each meal, in continuous cycles of five days on and five days off, half a teaspoonful of Formula 636 (available from the Heritage Store);
(27) take a good multiple vitamin/mineral supplement (or its equivalent) daily;
(28) avoid candy, cake, pies, pastries, and ice cream;
(29) try to drink six to eight glasses of water (preferably distilled) daily;
(30) avoid products containing vinegar (such as pickles, relish, and ketchup);
(31) have some gelatin with every meal (it aids absorption of nutrients);
(32) do not cook with condiments, including salt (it destroys much of the vitamin content of food);
(33) drink half a glass of warm water (preferably distilled) upon arising in the morning (it helps rid the body of toxins);

(34) take time to chew your food thoroughly (even liquids should be chewed two or three times before swallowing);

(35) take a digestive enzymes tablet with every meal;

(36) avoid products containing corn syrup;

(37) do not eat bananas unless vine ripened in your vicinity;

(38) have at least one leafy vegetable to every one of the pod variety;

(39) three times a day, *slowly* sip a teaspoonful of Campbell's Beef Broth (it helps confer strength and vitality); and

(40) once a day, take two or three heaping tablespoonfuls of Ovaltine (Malt Flavor) in a glass of skim milk, or drink an *MS Malt* (see page 71).

The preceding recommendations represent Plan "A" in the treatment of MS and pertain to *mild* cases in which there is no appreciable paralysis or disability – "just" the annoying signs and symptoms of the type listed on page 46.

TREATING CASES OF MODERATE SEVERITY (PLAN "B")

In treating cases of *moderate* severity (characterized by a significant degree of paralysis and disability but without total loss of the ability to ambulate), it is suggested that you adhere to Plan "A" with the following exceptions:

(1) increase the duration of the massage therapy session to forty minutes; and
(2) use the following ingredients in the wet cell battery:

(A) 2 pounds of copper sulfate,
(B) 4 ounces of sulfuric acid (33.33% solution),
(C) 7.1 grams of zinc particles, and
(D) 1/2 pound of willow charcoal.

TREATING SEVERE CASES (PLAN "C")

In treating *severe* cases of MS (characterized by extensive paralysis and disability with no ability to ambulate), it is suggested that you adhere to Plan "A" with the following exceptions:
(1) increase the duration of the massage therapy sessions to fifty minutes; and
(2) use the following ingredients in the wet cell battery:

(A) 2-1/2 pounds of copper sulfate,
(B) 4 ounces of sulfuric acid (41.75% solution),
(C) 8.8 grams of zinc particles, and
(D) 1/2 pound of willow charcoal.

DURATION OF TREATMENT

Treating multiple sclerosis using the Cayce approach is typically a long-term proposition. Depending on the severity of the condition, it could take up to seven years (or more) to achieve the maximum therapeutic effect (although definite signs of improvement should occur within the first 4 to 6 months).

WHAT I DID

In regard to the preceding treatment recommendations, I received massage therapy only sporadically (due to the expense and inconvenience involved), was sometimes remiss in following the dietary advice (due to a lack of self-control), chose the radial appliance as the vehicle for administering gold vibratorially (for reasons discussed in Chapter 5), and took a different approach to placing the copper electrode (for reasons discussed in Chapter 6).

CHAPTER 5

THE RELATIVE MERITS OF EACH APPLIANCE

THE WET CELL BATTERY

From all indications, the wet cell battery is clearly the "fast track" in terms of treating multiple sclerosis. It is the device recommended by the readings; it is the more powerful instrument; it does not depend on the body for its source of energy; and it is probably less sensitive to negative thoughts and emotions on the part of the person using it. It is undoubtedly the treatment of choice in most cases of multiple sclerosis.

THE RADIAL APPLIANCE

If you have a relatively mild, nonparalytic form of multiple sclerosis, you *might* – as I did – "get by" with the radial appliance. It can be very effective as a weapon in the arsenal of vibratory medicine, particularly if the person using it has chosen a "spiritual path" and is in general accord with its use. It is considerably less expensive to operate, especially on a long-term basis; there are no messy chemicals to mix periodically; when and if you finish using it to treat your MS, you can use it to your advantage *without* the solution jar; and you can even alternate its use both with and without the solution jar.

In my own case, I had consistently utilized the radial appliance for many years *without* the solution jar. Therefore, I was thoroughly familiar with its operation; my body was accustomed to the device; and I felt quite comfortable using it.

It was for the above reasons that I chose the radial appliance to treat my multiple sclerosis.

In retrospect, I believe that the wet cell battery would have produced more positive results more quickly, and, from that standpoint, would have been the better choice.

For persons at risk for developing MS (such as those with close relatives with the disease), the radial appliance might be an appropriate choice for use *prophylactically* (along the lines suggested in Chapter 7).

The radial appliance might also be a more appropriate choice in treating children and certain unusually sensitive individuals (who might find the wet cell battery too "harsh").

Trust in the LORD with all thine heart; and lean not unto thine own understanding. In all thy ways acknowledge him, and he shall direct thy paths.

Proverbs 3:5-6

CHAPTER 6

A WORD ABOUT ELECTRODE PLACEMENT

INTRODUCTION

In the practice of vibratory medicine, there are *two* main approaches to attaching the electrodes of either appliance to the body: the *general* and the *specific*.

THE GENERAL APPROACH

Regardless of which device you are using, if the nickel electrode is placed near the navel, and the copper electrode circulates around the extremities (as exemplified in Chapter 7), you are using the *general* approach.

This technique is particularly effective in the treatment of *widespread* conditions, such as systemic infections, and in the simultaneous treatment of *more than one* condition, such as multiple sclerosis and a heart problem.

This approach will probably *always* work to help alleviate *any* condition amenable to vibratory medicine. However, depending on the nature of the condition, it might take longer and be less effective than the specific approach.

In this technique, attachment of the copper electrode to the body is relatively easy to make, especially if – as in my case – you happen to be working *alone*.

It was for the above reasons that I chose the general approach in my use of the radial appliance.

This technique encompasses virtually all other variations of electrode placement.

Here, the attempt is made to focus *specifically* on a particular organ or system that is malfunctioning.

For example, in treating MS with the wet cell battery (as discussed in Chapter 4), you will notice that the electrodes are always placed in such a way that healing energies *must* flow through important nerve centers.

As another example, in treating certain female problems, the readings recommend placing the nickel electrode over the pubic area, and the copper electrode over the fourth lumbar vertebra. Here again, healing energies *must* bathe the affected organs.

This approach, however, usually works best in treating one problem at a time, and you may need the assistance of another person to *properly* place the copper electrode.

Seek ye the LORD while he may be found, call ye upon him while he is near.

Isaiah 55:6

CHAPTER 7

HOW I OVERCAME MS USING THE RADIAL APPLIANCE

INTRODUCTION

During the summer of 1991, I began to notice an occasional numbness in some of my fingers.

Unexplained muscle spasms and tremors also began to occur.

At times, I would be walking along on a smooth, flat surface and, for no apparent reason, stumble.

Occasionally, I would chew a bite of food, attempt to swallow it, and *nothing* would happen.

I was beginning to choke on fluids that "went down the wrong pipe."

My speech was becoming a little slurred.

Once in a while, my face would contort in an embarrassing and uncontrollable manner.

I was having trouble completely emptying my bladder.

Sometimes I would experience episodes of blurred vision, see flashes of light, and have an unscratchable itch behind my eyes.

My memory was beginning to fail.

I would often be unreasonably fatigued, inordinately depressed, and, on a few occasions, euphoric without cause.

During minor confrontations with co-workers, I tended to become almost hysterical.

My symptoms were aggravated by hot showers, heating pads and hot water bottles, hot environments, stress, viral infections, and, in particular, by a flu shot I received in the late fall of 1991.

It was obvious that I was developing a very serious and pervasive health problem.

It was *multiple sclerosis*.

THE REGIMEN THAT WORKED FOR ME

Based on my study of the Cayce readings, I decided to employ the radial appliance (beginning in November of 1991) in continuous cycles of 28 days (with a five day hiatus or "rest" interval between each cycle), using it with three ounces of gold chloride solution (in a concentration of one grain per ounce of distilled water) in the solution jar.

On *day one* of the cycle, I attached the copper electrode to the *inside* of my *right wrist* over the *radial artery*, which is the primary pulse point in the wrist (see Figure 1).

FIGURE 1:
ATTACHMENT OF THE COPPER ELECTRODE (WRIST).

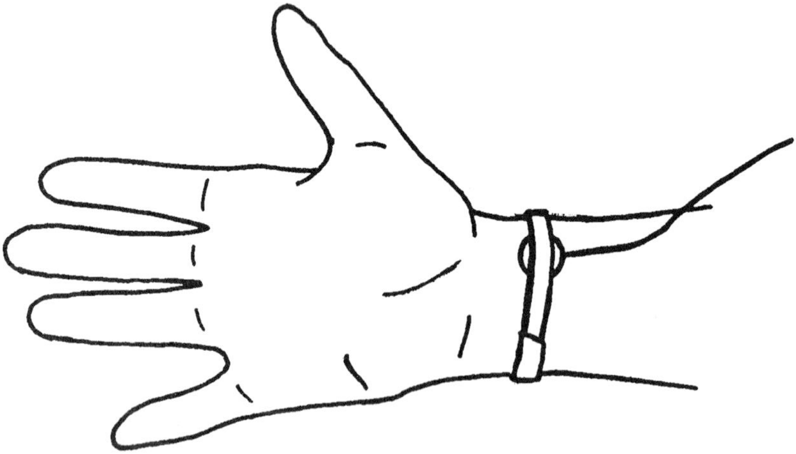

I applied the nickel electrode to my abdomen, *slightly above and to the right of my navel* (see Figure 2), putting a folded towel and pillow over it to keep it in place. Its application site was always the same for each day of the cycle (only the copper electrode changes position), and it represents the location of what the readings refer to as the "umbilical and lacteal duct plexus."

FIGURE 2:
ABDOMINAL PLACEMENT OF THE NICKEL ELECTRODE.

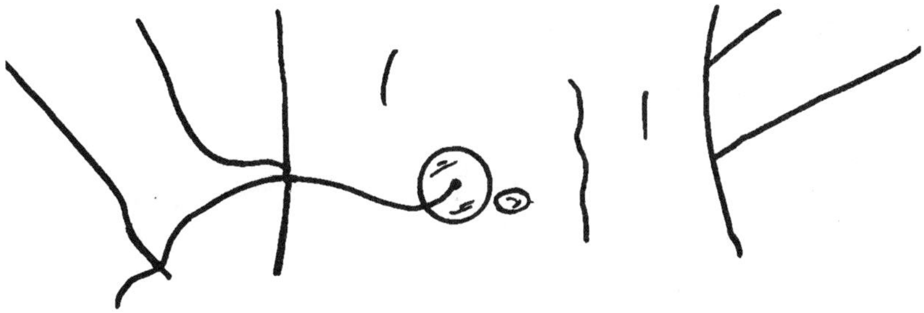

On *day two*, I attached the copper electrode over the radial artery in my *left wrist*.

On *day three*, I attached the copper electrode to the *inside* of my *left ankle* over the *posterior tibial artery*, which is the primary pulse point in the ankle (see Figure 3).

FIGURE 3:
ATTACHMENT OF THE COPPER ELECTRODE (ANKLE).

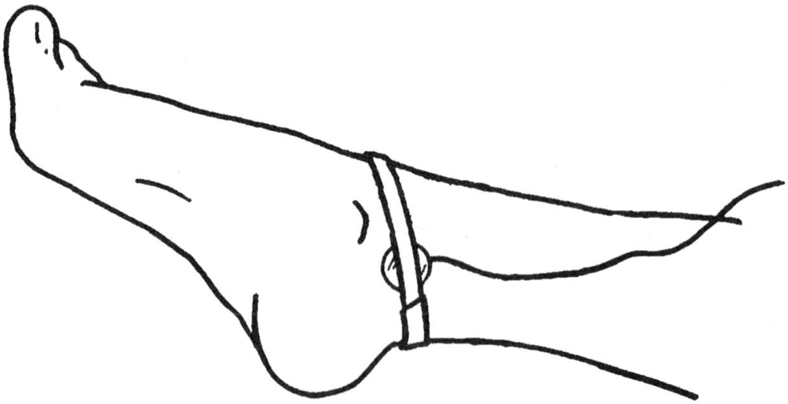

On *day four*, I attached the copper electrode to a comparable spot on my *right ankle*.

On *day five*, I placed the copper electrode on my *right wrist* again, and so on around each extremity for each day of the cycle.

At the end of the 28 day cycle, I would discontinue using the appliance for five days, after which I would repeat the cycle all over again.

TREATMENT RESULTS

I followed the above regimen faithfully – and continue to do so – and within a few months I began to experience considerably less fatigue. Within two years, all signs and symptoms of multiple sclerosis gradually disappeared and have not returned – *except* for brief periods during and/or following certain viral infections (such as Herpes simplex), unusually stressful situations, or when I have not kept up my treatments.

In my opinion, the basic cause of my condition (the inability of my body to properly assimilate gold) has not as yet been corrected, just compensated for. Perhaps, as I continue to employ vibratory medicine, maintain good dietary habits, etc., the basic cause will be eliminated, and I will be "cured." In the meantime, I am quite content to be "just" in a state of remission, and if that state should continue indefinitely, I should be equally content.

Some individuals who have utilized the *wet cell battery* appear to have achieved a cure. Jess Belcher, for example (cited in Chapter 8), no longer uses the wet cell, and her symptoms have not returned.

O taste and see that the LORD is good: blessed is the man that trusteth in him.

Psalm 34:8

CHAPTER 8

OVERCOMING MS USING THE WET CELL BATTERY

PHIL THOMAS' WET CELL THERAPY CENTER

Phil Thomas makes and sells the long pole version of the wet cell battery (which he believes is superior to the short pole version).

In 1993, he opened a wet cell therapy center in Virginia Beach for persons desiring to use the device.

He claims that a number of MS sufferers who came to the center experienced beneficial results.

One case in particular was that of Jess Belcher, who was diagnosed with MS at the age of 35.

Her symptoms included aching sensations in her legs, numbness on the left side of her body, losing her balance and falling, muscle spasms, headaches, and constant fatigue.

In addition to prayer, meditation, and dietary measures, she used the wet cell battery consistently for nine months.

She is now symptom-free and feeling fine. [1]

Another case was that of Maybritt Hansen, who was diagnosed with MS at the age of 37.

Her symptoms included tingling sensations, numbness, blurred and double vision, slurred speech, muscle weakness, poor coordination, muscle spasms, bladder and colon dysfunction, loss of balance, mental difficulties, severe fatigue, foot pain, hypertension, and paralysis.

---

[1] Deborah Seymour Taylor, "The Wet Cell Appliance," *Venture Inward*, July/August, 1993.

In addition to herbs, flower essences, gem elixirs, amino acids and other food supplements, she used the wet cell battery for four months, alternating between the use of gold chloride, silver nitrate, and spirits of camphor in the solution jar.

In just a matter of weeks, she reported her progress as "phenomenal." [2]

Still another case was that of Astrid Scammell, whose symptoms included incoordination, numbness, and foot pain.

After using the wet cell battery for a period of time, she reported a *marked* improvement in her condition. Even her digestion improved! [3]

Phil Thomas' phone number is listed in the Appendix.

OTHER WET CELL SUCCESS STORIES

Down through the years, *many* persons afflicted with multiple sclerosis have been helped with the wet cell battery, either working independently, under the care of a sympathetic healthcare professional, or under the auspices of such organizations as the A.R.E. Clinic in Phoenix, or the Scottsdale Holistic Medical Group in Scottsdale, Arizona.

---

[2] Maybritt Hansen, "The Wet Cell: Overcoming MS," *Venture Inward*, July/August, 1993.

[3] Deborah Seymour Taylor, "The Wet Cell Rediscovered," *Venture Inward*, May/June, 1994.

Tragically, very few of these success stories have been formally documented in books, magazines, or professional journals. Hopefully, in the not too distant future, as increasing numbers of people with MS realize the importance of documenting their experiences with vibratory medicine, that unfortunate situation will be rectified.

CHAPTER 9

QUESTIONS AND ANSWERS REGARDING THE APPLIANCES

1 (Q) Are the radial appliance and wet cell battery officially "approved" medical devices?

(A) No; I am sorry to say that they are not. To properly evaluate them would require very costly long-term, large-scale, controlled studies which, so far, no interested party has been financially equipped to undertake. With the exception of two small-scale studies (which demonstrated that the radial appliance used *without* the solution jar can (1) significantly improve peripheral circulation, and (2) measurably increase blood dopamine levels), about all that presently exists is a diverse group of people (like myself) who claim that they have been helped by the appliances in one way or another. Unfortunately, those are insufficient grounds for official approval.

2 (Q) What is the purchase price of each device?

(A) Currently, the average price of the radial appliance and the *short pole* version of the wet cell battery is under $200. The *long pole* version of the wet cell is proportionately more expensive.

3 (Q) Can improper use of either appliance be harmful?

(A) Definitely. As anyone in the healing arts can tell you – and the readings stress this fact, too – any therapeutic modality that has the potential for *good* also has the potential for *ill* if misapplied.

4 (Q) What does one do during the five day "rest" interval?

(A) Just live your life as usual – it is a rest from treatment, not from life!

5 (Q) Suppose I fall asleep while attached to the device and wake up an hour or two later?

(A) To prevent such occurrences, it is a good idea to purchase and utilize a timer.

6 (Q) Can I share the radial appliance with someone else?

(A) No. The readings specifically advised *against* that practice because, once you use the radial appliance, it becomes part of you – as personal an item as your toothbrush.

7 (Q) Can I share the wet cell battery with someone else?

(A) It is apparently permissible in most instances, but I advise against it.

8 (Q) Is attitude important in using the appliances?

(A) Very much so, particularly when using the radial appliance. If a person maintains a positive, hopeful, expectant attitude, keeping an open mind to real possibilities, and praying to God for healing and restoration, the appliances are likely to be much more effective than if one is filled with doubts, fear, and unbelief. Negative thoughts – as well as negative emotions like anger and resentment – seem to build a resistance that is difficult (if not impossible) for the appliances to overcome. Some readings on multiple sclerosis stated that *nothing* could be accomplished until and unless negativity – toward situations, circumstances, self, others, and God – was dealt with and eliminated.

9 (Q) What if I accidentally *drop* the radial appliance?

(A) I have dropped my unit several times on the bedroom rug and in the yard (although never on a really *hard* surface). It did not seem to harm the device, however, and I continue to use it to this day. Of course, if one or both terminals become damaged, the appliance will need repair or replacement.

10 (Q) Is there any way to "prove" that the radial appliance is working?

(A) Yes. The readings state that if the appliance is connected to an amputee, he or she will experience the presence of the lost limb. As far as I know, this test has never been performed.

11 (Q) Can I *recycle* the ice used with the radial appliance?

(A) Try to use a fresh batch each day. Small ice cubes are preferable to large ones, and *crushed* ice is better still.

12 (Q) Suppose the radial appliance does not receive any sun between treatments due to inclement weather or other causes?

(A) Use it anyway. Do *not* defer any treatments on that account. The same rule also applies if the wiring, electrodes, and loop of the wet cell battery do not receive any sun between treatments.

13 (Q) Should I discontinue using the device if I contract a cold, the flu, or some other infectious disease?

(A) If you are using gold chloride in the solution jar, the answer is "no." The readings suggest that administering gold vibratorially will help combat such infections. Once, for example, I developed a urinary tract infection. The bacteria causing it spread throughout my whole body and I developed septicemia. My temperature climbed at times to 103° F. To treat it, I used the radial appliance in the manner described in Chapter 7, ate light, nourishing meals (including quantities of lettuce), drank plenty of fluids (I found pineapple juice to be especially refreshing), took increased amounts of vitamin "C" and Formula 636, tried daily to work up a good sweat by walking (followed by a warm shower), gave myself an enema once a day after a bowel movement, took an occasional baby aspirin and employed an electric fan (to control my temperature), drank a cup of saffron tea at bedtime, and – of no less importance – prayed for my recovery. Within ten days, I was completely well. While an antibiotic (most likely a sulfonamide) could have been enlisted to treat this infection, I feared the potential adverse effects.

14 (Q) If vibratory medicine can be used to treat systemic infections, could it be used to treat AIDS?

(A) I would not be at all surprised if it were successful in at least *extending* and making *more bearable* the lives of those afflicted with the Human Immunodeficiency Virus. As suggested by the answer to the preceding question, however, vibratory medicine usually is most effectively utilized in conjunction with other therapies.

15 (Q) Is there any alternative to using the *lead* loop in the solution jar of the wet cell battery?

(A) Yes. Nickel and copper loops may also be used. They cost more, but last longer. Lead loops are preferable, however, because they present a larger surface area to the solution in the jar, are perhaps less chemically reactive to it, and were the type most frequently recommended by the readings.

16 (Q) Why is it necessary to *sand* the electrodes and the loop both before and after use?

(A) To insure that the device is functioning at top efficiency. You only want *bright metal* next to your skin and in the solution jar.

17 (Q) Should I sand the electrodes, the loop, and (if applicable) the poles even through brand new and unused?

(A) Absolutely. Just because these items are brand new does not guarantee that they are bright and shiny and clean.

18 (Q) How do I keep my *fingerprints* from getting on the electrodes and the loop?

(A) When you sand these items, I suggest you wear a pair of non-sterile, vinyl gloves (available from most surgical supply houses and pharmacies or by calling 1-800-BEDFORD).

19 (Q) How do I repair an electrode when I have sanded off thc hcad of thc pin to which thc wirc is attached?

(A) Take the electrode to the hardware store and locate a 3/8" long, round head bolt (steel for the nickel electrode and copper for the copper electrode) whose diameter is small enough to fit through the hole in the electrode vacated by the spent pin. Buy several bolts, because you will eventually need them. You will also need to buy two matching washers and a matching nut. Push the bolt through the hole in the electrode so that the head faces inward (that is, toward the body if it were in use). Put the two washers on the other end of the bolt and screw on the nut. Wrap about 3/8" of bare electrode wire around the bolt between the two washers. Tighten the nut, and you are back in business.

20 (Q) Should I keep a written record of my attachments to the device?

(A) Yes; unless you do, there will come a time when you cannot determine where to place the copper electrode, because you *forgot* where it was the day before.

21 (Q) Should I keep a written record of my use of the compound in the solution jar?

(A) Yes; that way, you will always know when to change it.

22 (Q) What if I attach myself to the device and then realize that I have incorrectly positioned the copper electrode?

(A) Simply remove the nickel electrode from the body, correctly reposition the copper electrode, and then reapply the nickel electrode.

23 (Q) Suppose, in my use of the radial appliance, I accidentally apply the *nickel* electrode first?

(A) Unlike the wet cell battery, the direction of energy flow when using the radial appliance depends on which electrode is *first* attached to the body. Applying the nickel electrode first will, as it were, throw the appliance into "reverse gear," causing energy to flow from the copper electrode, through the body, toward the nickel electrode. This is the *exact opposite* of what you want, and is of little or no therapeutic value. Skip the session for that day, and continue in the correct manner on the following day.

24 (Q) What if, *after* my session on the device, I realize that the copper electrode was incorrectly positioned?

(A) Just forget about it and try in your next session to proceed in the proper manner.

25 (Q) Suppose, as I am preparing to use the device, the electrodes accidentally *touch* each other?

(A) You have short-circuited the device. Skip the session for that day.

26 (Q) If I get the "urge" to reposition the nickel electrode slightly, is it permissible to do so?

(A) Yes; it is probably your body's way of telling you that it *needs* repositioning. The placement shown on page 49 is approximately correct for most individuals, but the *optimal* placement varies a little from person to person.

27 (Q) When is the best time of day to implement my treatment agenda?

(A) In the evening before retiring. If that is not feasible, try at least to schedule it for the *same* time every day.

28 (Q) Will I feel anything while attached to either appliance?

(A) Probably nothing definitive, except for an occasional feeling of nausea (in which case see below) or an occasional slight tingling sensation.

29 (Q) Will it ever be advisable to *cut short* my session on the device?

(A) Possibly. The thirty minute time limit specified in this publication is a good safe duration for most people to use most of the time. However, there may be occasions when your body is, for one reason or another, unprepared for a full session, and will so indicate by either an *increased pulse rate or a feeling of nausea.* Just discontinue that session and resume your regular treatment schedule on the following day. If it keeps recurring, however, you may need to shorten the planned duration of your daily sessions and gradually work up to the thirty minute mark.

CHAPTER 10

MISCELLANEOUS QUESTIONS AND ANSWERS

1 (Q) Was your condition ever officially diagnosed by a neurologist?

(A) No. As a healthcare professional, I am accustomed to attending to my *own* health needs. Therefore, I diagnosed it myself based on the many signs and symptoms I possessed which, in my opinion, were so characteristic of MS that no other diagnosis was reasonably possible. In addition, because I am a very private person, and because I did not care to be stigmatized as being afflicted with multiple sclerosis, I treated it myself, and have kept the whole matter a closely guarded secret – until now. By "coming out," I am hoping that *others* might benefit from my success with the Cayce approach to treating MS.

2 (Q) Do you eat foods that have a relatively high gold content?

(A) No. I do not make any special attempt to include them in my diet, nor do the readings on multiple sclerosis particularly recommend them. My need for gold is met by my use of the radial appliance.

3 (Q) What do the readings say about smoking?

(A) The readings say that smoking in *moderation* (three or four cigarettes a day) is not harmful.

However, they were referring to cigarettes devoid of additives or fillers, which are very difficult to obtain today. Besides, how many smokers do so in moderation? Edgar Cayce (who was not always successful in following his own readings) certainly did not, and it definitely shortened *his* life. Smoking killed my poor mother who, in the last days of her life, had to *fight* for every breath. Don't let that happen to you. *Don't smoke!*

4 (Q) What about water quality in this country?

(A) It is apparently much worse than most people realize. The readings advised drinking *boiled* water. In my opinion, due to pesticide runoff and other factors, the safest water to drink now is *distilled* (available at most pharmacies and supermarkets). Not all brands are of consistent quality, however. If it makes you thirsty or leaves an unpleasant aftertaste, try another brand.

5 (Q) Should I stay out of the sun?

(A) The Cayce readings advise avoiding direct sunlight between mid-morning and mid-afternoon. With the current depletion in the ozone layer, however, it might be wise to avoid direct exposure to the sun except during the early morning and late afternoon (unless you are wearing sunscreen and/or protective clothing). Sunlight is good for you, and you need it to be healthy. Just be careful *when* you get it!

6 (Q) Are there any exercises that would be helpful?

(A) According to the readings, *walking* (especially after dinner) is the *best* exercise (if need be, in a pattern of walk and rest, walk and rest); also good are *swimming*, and *stretching* (like a cat).

7 (Q) Do the readings give any advice about losing weight?

(A) Yes. In addition to eating along the lines suggested in Chapter 4, half an hour before each meal and at bedtime, drink a glass containing one ounce of distilled water to which three ounces of grape juice have been added. This simple concoction represents a natural appetite suppressant. It might also be a good idea to take a chromium picolinate tablet (available at most health food stores) on a daily basis. It apparently helps normalize blood glucose (sugar) levels, and studies suggest that most Americans are deficient in chromium.

8 (Q) Can you suggest a good *cleansing* diet?

(A) Yes. Eat nothing but raw, peeled Delicious apples for three days. During this period, drink nothing but distilled water. On the evening of the third day, take two tablespoonsful of olive oil. (If possible, obtain a colonic irrigation the next morning.) The readings claimed that this regimen would detoxify *any* system. It is probably wise to go on this diet *before* instituting *any* of the treatment recommendations suggested in this publication, and then again at least twice a year between cycles on the device and taking Formula 636.

9 (Q) Do you have any favorite *recipes*?

(A) Yes, these four:

(1) For breakfast, I usually have what you might call an "MS Malt." In preparing it,

(A) put two packets of artificial sweetener into an electric blender;

(B) add one envelope of Nonfat Dry Milk (which, when reconstituted, makes one quart);

(C) add two or three heaping tablespoonsful of Ovaltine (Malt Flavor);

(D) add one envelope of Knox Unflavored Gelatin;

(E) fill the blender with distilled water to the One Quart level; and

(F) cover and run the machine on low speed for about ten seconds.

(2) For lunch, I frequently eat an "egg yolk sandwich," which consists of one sliced hard-boiled egg yolk (sprinkled with gelatin) on whole wheat toast with lettuce and mayonnaise.

(3) For dinner, I often have "fish stew." To make it,

(A) put 10 ounces of frozen mixed vegetables into a stainless steel, porcelain, or glass pot;

(B) add 10 ounces of frozen chopped spinach;

(C) add one rounded tablespoonful of almonds;

(D) add one small sliced onion;

(E) add one sliced stick of celery;
(F) add 1/2 can of bean sprouts;
(G) add three tablespoonsful of juice from the can of bean sprouts;
(H) add 1-1/2 well-drained cans of tuna fish;
(I) add 1/4 cup of distilled water;
(J) cover and cook for forty-five minutes to an hour on medium-low heat;
(K) uncover and let cool for 20 minutes;
(L) mix in one envelope of Knox Unflavored Gelatin; and
(M) mix in one cup of unsweetened apple sauce.

(4) As a substitute for sipping teaspoonfuls of beef broth, I may sprinkle it over the top piece of toast on my egg yolk sandwich, and/or add it to my MS Malt.

10 (Q) How is it that, at the age of 58, you look so young?

(A) I believe the way in which I use the radial appliance makes of it a "fountain of youth." The readings claim that a person can almost *double* his or her life span by the vibratory administration of gold and silver. I do not use silver with the appliance, but apparently gold by itself is able to keep me "young looking."

11 (Q) Has the radial appliance helped your speech problem?

(A) When I was seven years old, I underwent emergency surgery to remove a badly inflamed appendix. The whole experience was so upsetting and traumatic that I began to stutter. I believe that my use of the appliance has significantly improved my verbal fluency, but the problem is still there, and I still have difficulty expressing myself now and then, depending on the situation.

12 (Q) Has the radial appliance helped your nervousness?

(A) When I was a toddler, I accidentally ingested some arsenic ant poison. Fortunately, I received the antidote in time to prevent a fatal outcome. Even so, the poison left me a somewhat nervous individual and, although the appliance has definitely helped in that regard, I still have an occasional problem with facial tics.

13 (Q) Apart from the radial appliance and wet cell battery, is there any other way to administer substances vibratorially?

(A) Yes and no. At the time the readings were given, there was a device produced commercially known as the "B" battery. It was used to help power the vacuum tubes in radio equipment.

A number of readings (including one on MS) recommended it as a tool of vibratory medicine. It was very convenient to use because, unlike the radial appliance, it did not require the handling of ice and, unlike the wet cell battery, it did not require the mixing of chemicals. Unfortunately, it went out of production many years ago. Perhaps some enterprising company or individual will resurrect it, as plans and specifications for it must exist *somewhere*. Also, it is possible that one or more (or a combination) of the myriad batteries presently available would suffice as a vehicle for vibratory medicine – an intriguing question which, hopefully, will be addressed and resolved by future research.

14 (Q) Is there any tangible evidence to suggest that the *liver* is involved in the etiology of multiple sclerosis?

(A) Yes. There tends to be a *hardening* of the ductal system associated with the gall bladder (predisposing the gall bladder to infection) and of that portion of the liver surrounding the hepatic duct.

15 (Q) What is the chief *drawback* of vibratory medicine?

(A) Its slowness, particularly in treating neurological problems like multiple sclerosis. It would seem that a number of individuals who received readings for MS became impatient, discouraged, and discontinued treatment prematurely. That is why the readings often advised *patience and persistence* in its application.

16 (Q) What are my chances of recovery if I employ vibratory medicine?

(A) Most regrettably, there are no studies, no research results, and thus no hard data upon which to base a prognosis. My own personal feeling in the matter is that if you faithfully and conscientiously follow the treatment recommendations outlined in Chapter 4, your chances of experiencing at least *some* improvement in your condition – if not total recovery – are good to excellent. Bear in mind, however, that it may take *years* to fully reap the benefits of this endeavor.

17 (Q) Are there any *contraindications* to the use of vibratory medicine?

(A) Do *not* employ vibratory medicine if you

(1) are pregnant,
(2) are angry or upset,
(3) have alcohol in your system, or
(4) have just taken a dose of atomidine.

18 (Q) What is atomidine?

(A) An aqueous solution of iodine trichloride. When used full strength, it is effective as an antiseptic in treating minor cuts and abrasions. It can also be used in the solution jar of either appliance, and several readings recommended that it be alternated with gold chloride and/or other compounds in the treatment of multiple sclerosis. Greatly diluted, it can be taken by mouth to treat not only iodine deficiency states, but also (according to the readings) Ménière's disease, myasthenia gravis, various glandular problems, and a number of other conditions for which iodine has not as yet been recognized as being of therapeutic value. In several cases of MS, the readings recommended taking atomidine by mouth, but *not* just prior to implementing vibratory medicine.

19 (Q) Should I include atomidine in my treatment of MS?

(A) Formula 636 (recommended in Chapter 4) contains atomidine (in addition to ginseng, liver extract, and other helpful ingredients).

20 (Q) Where did the information in the readings come from?

(A) The source varied depending on the type of information being sought. In the case of the "physical" readings, Edgar Cayce visited "in spirit" the person for whom the reading was being given, performed a complete examination, determined the nature of the problem, ascertained the most appropriate treatment recommendations, and perhaps (as an aside) commented on the weather or soil conditions where the recipient of the reading happened to be living. When he awoke, he would have no recollection of this "visit," nor of anything said during the course of the reading.

21 (Q) How was Edgar Cayce able to perform this incredible feat?

(A) That is a question that can perhaps best be answered by the angel mentioned in Chapter 1.

22 (Q) What is your relationship to the Association for Research and Enlightenment?

(A) I am a Life Member of the A.R.E. and have been a student of the Cayce readings for over thirty-five years. The information in the readings has helped me *greatly*, not only in terms of defeating multiple sclerosis, but in many lesser ways as well. In fact, it is safe to say that I owe my life to the readings.

23 (Q) Why do MS symptoms tend to worsen in relation to heat, stress, viral infections and vaccinations against them?

(A) Some of the symptoms of multiple sclerosis (such as dry mouth, tremors, blurred vision, urinary retention, and constipation) are due to a relative *increase* in innervation from the *sympathetic* division of the autonomic nervous system (as innervation from the central nervous system becomes progressively less dominant). The effect of heat, stress, viral infections and vaccinations against them is to cause a *further* increase in sympathetic innervation, thus potentiating these symptoms. Moreover, some viruses and their vaccines exert a direct or indirect *neurotoxic* effect. The combination of doubly increased sympathetic innervation *plus* neurotoxicity can aggravate (or cause to surface) a wide range of MS symptoms.

24 (Q) Why do antiviral drugs seem to help multiple sclerosis?

(A) By inhibiting viral infections, they tend to eliminate *that* source of increased sympathetic innervation and possible neurotoxicity.

25 (Q) Is there any *drugless* way to decrease heightened levels of sympathetic innervation and thereby reduce some symptoms associated with MS?

(A) Vibratory medicine represents a long-term solution to the problem. As a temporary palliative measure, you might try taking (as directed on the label) Passion Flower Fusion (available from the Heritage Store). It is a natural sympatholytic, relaxant, and anticonvulsant. The readings often recommended it in cases of epilepsy as a non-habit forming substitute for Dilantin and phenobarbital. It may also be helpful in curbing the muscle spasms associated with spinal cord injuries.

26 (Q) In treating MS, does the vibratory administration of gold have any effect other than eliminating the lack of that mineral in the system?

(A) Yes. It also promotes *central nervous system regeneration*. For that reason, the readings very often suggested its use in treating neurological problems totally unrelated to gold deficiency states, such as Down's syndrome, polio, stroke, and spinal cord injuries.

27 (Q) Is it possible to *overdose* on gold administered vibratorially?

(A) Definitely. You may become headachy, develop a bad taste in your mouth, and experience other unpleasant reactions. To avoid this occurrence, be sure to stay within the parameters of vibratory medicine specified in this book.

28 (Q) Do any readings on MS recommend taking gold by mouth instead of (or in addition to) vibratorially?

(A) Yes, several. Apparently, in these cases, the gold deficiency was diet related, or at least could be helped by an oral gold supplement.

29 (Q) Can you recommend a good laxative?

(A) Yes, Zilatone (available from the Heritage Store). One tablet (taken between meals or, preferably, at bedtime) will not only promote a good bowel movement, but will also stimulate the functioning of the liver (which, in cases of multiple sclerosis, is especially desirable). Like most laxatives, it also makes a rather good headache remedy (for many headaches stem from adverse conditions in the gastrointestinal tract). You should have at least *one* bowel movement daily, even if it requires giving yourself an enema.

30 (Q) If only the vibration of a substance (and not the actual substance itself) is transmitted into the body via vibratory medicine, how is it beneficial?

(A) My impression from the readings is that one or a combination of the following mechanisms may be at work in any given situation: (1) the body responds as if the necessary substance(s) were physically present, (2) the body is stimulated to create the necessary substance(s), or (3) the body is encouraged to increase assimilation of the necessary substance(s). In the case of MS, I believe the latter mechanism predominates.

31 (Q) Does *childbearing* put a woman at risk for developing MS?

(A) Yes. Depending on the circumstances, pregnancy can leave a woman *nutritionally bankrupt* and with certain glands that are *spent*. That occurrence, coupled with an MS predisposition, can trigger the condition. The prevalence of multiple sclerosis among young mothers just starting a family can be explained in this way.

32 (Q) Why do MS symptoms seem to abate during pregnancy and menstruation?

(A) The glandular disturbance associated with the genesis of multiple sclerosis appears to be at least partially corrected or offset during such periods.

33 (Q) What is one of the best ways to *prevent* MS?

(A) Adhering to the dietary advice in Chapter 4.

34 (Q) What about bee venom therapy?

(A) It was not mentioned in the readings on MS and, in my opinion, although it may afford symptomatic relief in some cases, it neither addresses the cause of the disease, nor can it reverse the attendant neurological damage.

35 (Q) Why is MS more prevalent in some geographical regions?

(A) Some of the factors responsible may include variations in dietary habits, the presence of environmental toxins (especially mercury), genetic differences among groups of people, the lack of sunlight, and the ready availability of nutritionally deficient food (grown on depleted soil, milled, processed, and refined).

36 (Q) Why do women develop MS at a rate more than double that of men?

(A) I believe it is because women are more susceptible to glandular disturbances, are more prone to develop vertebral subluxations (due to greater joint laxity), and are more likely to be nutritionally compromised (due to relatively poorer diet, monthly iron loss, and the nutritional demands of pregnancy).

37 (Q) Why is muscle pain a symptom in some cases of multiple sclerosis?

(A) It may be related to the attempt on the part of muscle tissue to "wrest," so to speak, necessary nutrients from the surrounding circulation.

38 (Q) Should I have my fillings replaced, as some recommend?

(A) You may if you wish, but, since the readings never recommended that procedure in the treatment of MS, it is apparently unnecessary.

39 (Q) Besides vibratory medicine, diet, and massage, is there any other therapy that might help?

(A) Yes. Osteopathic spinal manipulation was recommended in enough readings on multiple sclerosis (about 1 in 4) that you might consider obtaining (on a twice per week basis) a series of 6 to 8 full-spine manipulations – including the sacrum and coccyx – *before* initiating your first vibratory medicine cycle, and periodically thereafter. Unfortunately, very few osteopathic physicians currently practice spinal manipulation, so you may need to do some calling around to find a suitable practitioner.

40 (Q) What if vibratory medicine does not work for me?

(A) It is known that some individuals do not respond to vibratory medicine. Even so, if there has been absolutely no improvement in your condition after the first several months of treatment (assuming you were following all procedures correctly, your device was functioning properly, and all connections were good), consider making the following changes in the treatment plan:

(1) if you were using the radial appliance, try the wet cell battery;

(2) if you were using the short pole version of the wet cell, try the long pole version;

(3) if you were using the general approach to electrode placement, try the specific approach;
(4) if you were following Plan "A," try Plan "B;"
(5) if you were following Plan "B," try Plan "C;"
(6) increase the dosage of Formula 636 to one teaspoonful after each meal;
(7) if you have not already done so, obtain the osteopathic spinal manipulations mentioned in the answer to the preceding question;
(8) strive to rid yourself of all anger, resentment, bitterness, unforgiveness, prejudice, hatred, animosity, jealousy, hostility, unbelief in the efficacy of vibratory medicine, and all other negative attitudes and emotions;
(9) above all, get right with God by sending for, listening to, and heeding the counsel contained on the "Unshackled!" tape mentioned on page 116;
(10) other options include increasing the duration of your vibratory medicine sessions, increasing both the size of the solution jar and the amount of solution, increasing the concentration of the solution, decreasing the length of the "rest" interval, and alternating gold chloride with commercial strength spirits of

camphor and/or a 2% solution of silver nitrate. See the readings on MS for examples of these and other possibilities.

41 (Q) Do you havc any additional helpful advice?

(A) Yes. If you have not already done so, call the Multiple Sclerosis Foundation (1-800-441-7055), the Multiple Sclerosis Association of America (1-800-833-4672), and the National Multiple Sclerosis Society (1-800-344-4867) to obtain information regarding the many useful publications and services available from these organizations to persons with MS. Also, get plenty of sleep, and avoid stress, heat, viral infections, and overexertion.

42 (Q) What do you foresee as the future of vibratory medicine?

(A) As research focused on vibratory medicine goes forward, and as its value in treating a wide range of conditions becomes increasingly evident, I believe that, in time to come, every major hospital and medical center will have – in addition to departments of massage therapy and manual medicine (spinal manipulation) – a Department of Vibratory Medicine, particularly those institutions engaged in the care and treatment of persons afflicted not only with multiple sclerosis, but also with spinal cord injuries, postpolio syndrome, muscular dystrophy, mental retardation, Alzheimer's disease, Parkinson's disease, Lou Gehrig's disease, and other currently incurable neuromuscular/neuropsychiatric disorders. Textbooks will be written on the subject; it will be taught in medical and other healthcare programs; and some healthcare professionals will specialize in it. Eventually, it may even be hailed as one of the greatest contributions to modern medicine since the advent of penicillin.

43 (Q) While we are on the subject of foreseeing the future, do the readings predict when Jesus will return?

(A) 1998.

AFTERWORD

It has been said that the longest journey begins with the first step. Please do not be deterred by the protracted nature of the Cayce approach to overcoming multiple sclerosis. For, in my opinion, in the present state of our knowledge, there *is* no better alternative.

Therefore, do not delay!

The time to begin is now!

It is much easier for vibratory medicine to *halt* the progress of MS than – after the damage has been done – to *reverse* it. So, even if you cannot follow *all* the suggestions outlined in this book (such as receiving massage therapy after each vibratory medicine session), implement as much of the program as possible. Partial compliance with the Cayce regimen is far better than total noncompliance. You *owe* it to yourself *and* to your loved ones.

Vibratory medicine may not work in every case, but it works often enough that it should be *tried* in every case – and that includes *yours*.

And may God be with you!

APPENDIX

SOURCES OF INFORMATION AND SUPPLY

The radial appliance and wet cell battery (and their various solutions, chemicals, and accessories) are presently available from a number of suppliers, including:

(1) The Heritage Store (1-800-862-2923),
(2) The A.R.E. Bookstore (757-428-3588, ext. 7231),
(3) The A.R.E. Press (1-888-273-0050),
(4) The A.R.E. Clinic (602-955-0551),
(5) The Scottsdale Holistic Medical Group (602-990-1528),
(6) Bruce Barr (1-800-269-2502),
(7) Tom Dewey (1-888-590-7058),
(8) Phil Thomas (757-422-8513), and
(9) Tom Hildebrand (919-742-3379).

In general, due to the currently unproven nature and value of the appliances, none of the above parties make any medical claims regarding them.

Additional information about the appliances may be obtained from the above sources, as well as from the A.R.E. Library (757-428-3588, ext. 7141), and the A.R.E. Circulating Files Department (1-800-333-4499).

Home Health Products (1-800-284-9123) supplies some of the *other* items mentioned in this publication (such as Formula 636), as does the Heritage Store, the A.R.E. Bookstore, the A.R.E. Clinic, and the Scottsdale Holistic Medical Group.

BIBLIOGRAPHY

Barr, B., *Compilation of Readings on Multiple Sclerosis*, Downington: Barr Products, Inc.

Barr, B., *The Radiac Book*, Downington: Barr Products, Inc.

Cayce, E.E., *Two Electrical Appliances Described in the Edgar Cayce Readings*, Virginia Beach: The A.R.E. Press, 1993

Delany, D., "Glutamate Gloom," *Healthways*, June, 1976

Delany, D., "New Hope for Headache Sufferers," *Health World*, Winter, 1986/87

Delany, D., "An Alternative Therapy: Vibratory Gold," *Virginia Nurses Today*, July/August/September, 1997

DeMarco, T., "Favorable Results in Field Test of the Impedance Device," *Venture Inward*, May/June, 1989

Frankel, D., *Living with MS*, New York: The National Multiple Sclerosis Society, 1994

Grady, H., "The Cayce Impedance Device: A Gift on the Doorstep," *Venture Inward*, May/June, 1989

Hansen, M., "The Wet Cell: Overcoming MS," *Venture Inward*, July/August, 1993

Karp, R.A., *Edgar Cayce Encyclopedia of Healing*, New York: Warner Books, 1986

Mabery, M.V., *Inner Cycles of Health: Living with Multiple Sclerosis,* Waldorf: 21st Century Online Publishing, 1996

McGarey, W.A., *Physician's Reference Notebook*, Virginia Beach: The A.R.E. Press, 1983

McMillin, D., and Richards, D.G., *The Radial Appliance and the Wet Cell Battery*, Virginia Beach: Lifeline Press, 1994

Pahnke, W.N., *Multiple Sclerosis Research Bulletin*, Virginia Beach: The Edgar Cayce Foundation, 1990

Parisen, B., and B., "Our Experiences with the Radio-Active Appliance," *The A.R.E. Journal*, March, 1978

Reilly, H.J., and Brod, R.H., *The Edgar Cayce Handbook for Health Through Drugless Therapy*, New York: Macmillan Pub. Co., 1975

Richards, D.G., "The Radio-Active Appliance Really Works," *Venture Inward*, March/April, 1996

Rowland, L.P., editor, *Merritt's Textbook of Neurology*, 9th edition, Philadelphia: Williams & Wilkins, 1995

Stearn, J., *Edgar Cayce – The Sleeping Prophet,* New York: Bantam Books, 1967

Sugrue, T., *The Story of Edgar Cayce – There is a River*, Virginia Beach: The A.R.E. Press, 1973

Taylor, D.S., "The Wet Cell Appliance," *Venture Inward*, July/August, 1993

Taylor, D.S., "The Wet Cell Rediscovered," *Venture Inward*, May/June, 1994

Turner, G.D., and St. Clair, M.G., *Individual Reference File of Extracts from the Edgar Cayce Readings*, Virginia Beach: The Edgar Cayce Foundation, 1976

Wagner, K., "Alternative MS Treatment Works For Therapist," *Port Folio*, April 1, 1997

Wolfenden, A., "There *Is* Hope For MS," *Dimensions*, June, 1996

Copies of most of the *books* listed in this section may be purchased from either the Heritage Bookstore (1-800-862-2923) or the A.R.E. Bookstore (757-428-3588, ext. 7231).

Copies of most of the *articles* listed in this section may be purchased from the A.R.E. Library (757-428-3588, ext. 7141).

To order a video of A&E's biography of Edgar Cayce, call 1-800-423-1212.

INDEX

A

B

C

I

J

N

O

P

Q

R

S

T

W

Y

Z

ABOUT
THE
AUTHOR

Dr. Dudley Delany is a retired chiropractor, massage therapist, and registered nurse. He is also a born-again Christian whose testimony was broadcast world-wide in 1974 on the dramatic radio series, "Unshackled!"* He currently resides in Hampton, Virginia, where he is actively engaged in spreading the good news about vibratory medicine.

The author *welcomes* your questions, comments, and suggestions. Please direct your correspondence to him in care of the publisher.

---

*To obtain a cassette tape of this broadcast, send $3.00, together with a request for program number 1220, to: The Pacific Garden Mission, Chicago, IL 60605.

ORDER FORM

Meridian Publications
P.O. Box 7987
Hampton, VA 23666

Please send me_______ copies of **The Edgar Cayce Way of Overcoming Multiple Sclerosis: Vibratory Medicine** at $10.95 per copy. I have included $3.50 for shipping and handling. (Virginia residents, please add 4 1/2% sales tax.) Enclosed is my check or money order for $ ___________ .

Name (please print) ___________________________

Address _____________________________________

City ____

State _______________________________________

Zip Code ____________________________________

Thank you for your order.

SATISFACTION GUARANTEED OR YOUR MONEY REFUNDED!

For God so loved the world, that he gave his only begotten Son, that whosoever believeth in him should not perish, but have everlasting life.

John 3:16

ORDER FORM

Meridian Publications
P.O. Box 7987
Hampton, VA 23666

Please send me_______ copies of **The Edgar Cayce Way of Overcoming Multiple Sclerosis: Vibratory Medicine** at $10.95 per copy. I have included $3.50 for shipping and handling. (Virginia residents, please add 4 1/2% sales tax.) Enclosed is my check or money order for $ ___________ .

Name (please print) ____________________________

Address ____________________________________

City _______________________________________

State ______________________________________

Zip Code ___________________________________

Thank you for your order.

SATISFACTION GUARANTEED OR YOUR MONEY REFUNDED!

For God so loved the world, that he gave his only begotten Son, that whosoever believeth in him should not perish, but have everlasting life.

John 3:16